HERBAL REMEDIES FOR VULVODYNIA AND PELVIC PAIN

Empower Your Healing Journey With Herbal Solutions For Lasting Wellness, Restoring Comfort And Well-Being

DR. CARDEN KYRIE

DISCLAIMER

The only goal of this book is informational. Every effort has been taken by the author and publisher to ensure that the information provided is accurate. But the material in this book is given "as is," without any express or implied representation, warranty, or condition as to its accuracy, completeness, or suitability for any particular purpose.

Any loss, damage, or injury resulting from using the information in this book, or from any action or decision made as a result of such use, will not be covered by the author's or publisher's liability. It is recommended that readers seek the assistance of a certified specialist for guidance specific to their situation.

The opinions and viewpoints conveyed in this book belong to the author and may not necessarily represent the official stance or policies of any specified organizations or people. Any likeness to real-life occurrences, places, or people—living or deceased—is wholly coincidental.

No specific product, service, or therapy discussed in this book is endorsed by the author or publisher. Any reference to goods or services is made only for informative reasons and is not intended as a recommendation or endorsement.

Before making any judgments or acting on any information, readers are urged to independently confirm it all. Any unfavorable effects or repercussions arising from the usage of the material included in this book are disclaimed by the author and publisher.

By using this book, you consent to absolving the publisher and author of any and all claims, obligations, or losses resulting from your use of the material in it.

I appreciate your cooperation and understanding.

TABLE OF CONTENTS

CHAPTER ONE

INTRODUCTION TO VULVODYNIA AND PELVIC PAIN

AN OVERVIEW OF PELVIC PAIN AND VULVODYNIA

A complicated and frequently misdiagnosed medical illness, vulvodynia is a chronic pain syndrome that affects the vulva and has a substantial influence on the lives of individuals who suffer from it. The external genitalia, or vulva, can develop hypersensitivity, which results in chronic pain and discomfort. In addition to being physically demanding, this illness can have a significant emotional and psychological impact on people. Investigating the complex network of variables that lead to vulvodynia's emergence and the difficulties in diagnosing and treating it are essential to comprehend the condition.

A prevalent issue that impacts people of all ages and genders is pelvic pain, which is a more general phrase for discomfort in the pelvic area. The bladder, intestines, and reproductive organs are among the important organs located in the pelvic region. Numerous conditions, including gastrointestinal diseases and gynecological concerns, can cause pain in this area. A comprehensive approach to treating pelvic pain necessitates an accurate diagnosis and successful therapy due to the wide range of probable causes.

Examining the field of vulvodynia and pelvic discomfort highlights the significance of treating patients holistically, utilizing methods outside traditional medical approaches. Natural therapies—which rely on lifestyle changes, herbal treatments, and alternative therapies—have garnered recognition as supplemental approaches to treating various ailments. Acknowledging the limitations of traditional treatments and the possible advantages of implementing a more patient-centered and integrative approach is necessary to appreciate the significance of natural remedies.

THE VALUE OF NATURAL TREATMENTS

Natural therapies are significant when it comes to vulvodynia and pelvic discomfort because of their potential for effectiveness as well as their capacity to lessen adverse effects that are frequently connected to pharmaceutical solutions. Because of worries about the side effects of long-term pharmaceutical use, many people are looking for alternate solutions. Herbal supplements, food changes, and physical therapy are examples of natural remedies that provide a kinder and more long-lasting method of managing symptoms.

Moreover, the comprehensive approach of natural therapies corresponds with the knowledge that pelvic pain and vulvodynia frequently have multiple underlying causes. These diseases can be exacerbated by psychological causes, hormone imbalances, and musculoskeletal problems, which calls for an all-encompassing approach to treatment. Natural treatments promote a more comprehensive sense of well-being by addressing not only the physical symptoms but also the emotional and mental parts of the pain experience.

This examination of vulvodynia and pelvic discomfort highlights the need for a comprehensive knowledge of these illnesses to provide appropriate treatment. The treatment paradigm's integration of natural therapies is a reflection of a larger movement in healthcare toward patient-centered, individualized care. The use of complementary therapies is a viable path toward better results and a higher standard of living for individuals dealing with vulvodynia and pelvic pain as medical professionals continue to explore the intricacies of these difficult conditions.

CHAPTER TWO

KNOWLEDGE OF VULVODYNIA

TYPES AND DEFINITION

A complicated and sometimes misdiagnosed medical illness called vulvodynia is defined by persistent pain in the vulvar region, which encompasses a woman's external genital organs. Generally speaking, vulvodynia discomfort is characterized as a burning, stinging, or stabbing feeling that can happen on its own or be brought on by certain behaviors like extended sitting or sexual activity. In addition to having a substantial negative influence on a woman's quality of life, this illness can cause emotional discomfort and sexual dysfunction.

Vulvodynia comes in different forms, each with unique traits. The most prevalent kind of vulvodynia, known as localized vulvodynia, is typified by pain in a particular vulva location that is frequently brought on by pressure or touch.

Widespread pain across the vulvar region without a known reason is known as generalized vulvodynia. Provoked vestibulodynia is a different kind in which the pain is localized at the vaginal entrance and is usually brought on by pressure or touch, like during intercourse.

Since the precise causes of vulvodynia are unknown, diagnosing and treating the ailment can be difficult. Vulvodynia can arise as a result of several reasons, including inflammation, hormone fluctuations, hereditary susceptibility, and abnormalities in the vulva's nerve fibers.

In certain instances, a history of recurring vaginal infections or persistent yeast infections may also be relevant. Moreover, psychological elements like stress and anxiety might make symptoms worse.

REASONS AND DANGER ELEMENTS

A higher probability of having vulvodynia has been linked to several risk factors. Women who have experienced various pain conditions or chronic pelvic discomfort in the past may be more vulnerable. Moreover, a history of sexual abuse or trauma is seen as a possible risk factor. Vulvodynia may also result from hormonal changes, such as those that happen after menopause, pregnancy, or when using specific birth control techniques.

TYPICAL SYMPTOMS

Vulvodynia can cause a wide range of symptoms, but frequent ones include increased sensitivity to touch, discomfort during sexual activity, and a persistent burning or stabbing sensation. The discomfort might affect a woman's regular activities, such as sitting for long periods or exercising, and it can be either continuous or sporadic.

To diagnose vulvodynia, it is frequently necessary to rule out other possible reasons for vulvar pain, such as infections or skin disorders. To make a diagnosis, a thorough medical history, a pelvic exam, and occasionally specialist testing may be performed. Individualized treatment plans may combine medicinal, physical, and psychological therapy to address vulvodynia. For those with vulvodynia, medication, physical therapy, and cognitive-behavioral therapy are frequently used to treat symptoms and enhance general well-being.

CHAPTER THREE

PELVIC PAIN: ITS ORIGINS AND EFFECTS

RECOGNIZING VARIOUS PELVIC PAIN TYPES

Complex and multidimensional, pelvic pain can significantly affect a person's day-to-day functioning. The wide variety of possible causes of pelvic pain presents one of the difficulties in treating it; therefore, proper identification is essential to efficient treatment. There are several forms of pelvic pain, each with unique traits and underlying causes.

Pelvic discomfort is frequently caused by endometriosis, a condition in which tissue resembling the lining of the uterus grows outside the uterus. This may result in severe discomfort, scarring, and inflammation during the menstrual cycle. Pelvic inflammatory disease (PID) is another common reason; it is frequently brought on by STDs that damage the reproductive organs and cause pain and discomfort.

Pelvic pain can also be caused by musculoskeletal conditions, such as dysfunction of the pelvic floor. Dysfunction in the pelvic floor muscles can result in persistent pain, and these muscles are essential in maintaining the pelvic organs. Furthermore, pelvic pain may be a symptom of disorders such as interstitial cystitis and irritable bowel syndrome (IBS), underscoring the interdependence of many body systems.

EFFECTS ON DAY-TO-DAY LIVING

Pelvic pain has a significant impact on day-to-day functioning, influencing both physical and mental health. People who suffer from persistent pelvic pain frequently find it difficult to carry out daily tasks including working, exercising, and interacting with others. The ongoing agony might set off a vicious cycle that makes the pain worse by causing weariness, disturbed sleep, and increased stress.

Furthermore, it's important to recognize the psychological toll that pelvic pain can have. Anxiety and despair may be exacerbated by the chronic nature of the illness and the uncertainty surrounding it. As people deal with the difficulties of controlling pelvic discomfort, relationships may also become strained, affecting social interactions as well as personal relationships.

CONNECTION BETWEEN PELVIC PAIN AND VULVODYNIA

It is important to understand that vulvodynia is a particular subtype of pelvic pain that concentrates on discomfort or pain in the vulvar region when examining the association between vulvodynia and pelvic pain. This ailment is characterized by burning, stinging, or irritation. There is a complex link between this condition and more general pelvic pain. Because vulvar discomfort can cause stress and dysfunction in the pelvic floor muscles, which in turn can exacerbate general pelvic pain, vulvodynia may be a contributing factor to a cycle of pelvic pain.

The interaction between pelvic discomfort and vulvodynia highlights the necessity of a thorough and interdisciplinary approach to diagnosis and care. For successful treatment and an enhanced quality of life, pelvic pain must be addressed on the physical, emotional, and relationship levels. Through an understanding of the many forms of pelvic pain and its effects, medical professionals can customize interventions to meet the unique requirements of patients dealing with this difficult condition.

CHAPTER FOUR
TRADITIONAL INTERVENTIONS
MEDICAL METHODS

Medical approaches cover a wide range of therapies intended to cure different medical diseases. Medication, physical therapy, and even surgical procedures are part of these methods. The type and severity of the ailment, in addition to the specifics of each patient, will determine the course of treatment.

DRUGS

In traditional medical procedures, medications are essential. They are intended to treat infections, control chronic illnesses, or lessen symptoms. Prescription meds are for more serious diseases, while over-the-counter drugs are for milder ones. The goal of the pharmacological approach is to restore normal physiological activities by using medications to target certain pathways, receptors, or microbes within the body.

PHYSICAL MEDICINE

Another important part of traditional therapies is physical therapy, especially for musculoskeletal and rehabilitative conditions. Physical therapists use a range of methods, exercises, and modalities to increase function, lessen pain, and improve mobility. This method is frequently used to treat ailments like back discomfort, joint injuries, and post-operative recuperation. The goal of physical therapy is to improve the body's inherent healing abilities through non-invasive techniques.

SURGICAL TECHNIQUES

A more intrusive but occasionally required component of traditional medical therapies is surgical procedures. When other treatments are found to be insufficient or when a condition needs to be treated right away, surgery is frequently taken into consideration. Surgical methods vary based on the complexity of the medical problem; they can involve minor procedures or big operations. Tumor excision, organ transplants, joint replacements, and corrective surgery for anatomical defects are common indications for surgical treatments.

CONSTRAINTS AND ADVERSE REACTIONS

Medical techniques, while beneficial, are not without restrictions and potential negative effects. Each modality has these. Despite helping treat symptoms, medications might have unfavorable side effects, combine with other drugs, or lead to dependence problems. Despite being widely regarded as safe, physical therapy may not be able to treat all diseases or offer quick relief. Some patients find surgical treatments less appealing due to the dangers involved, including infections, problems, and lengthy recovery times.

Furthermore, the efficacy of these traditional treatments varies from patient to patient, underscoring the necessity of individualized medical care. Healthcare providers frequently carefully evaluate the patient's medical history, preferences, and the particulars of the ailment they are treating before selecting one of these modalities.

The foundation of contemporary healthcare is comprised of traditional medical techniques such as prescription drugs, physical rehabilitation, and surgery. Even though these techniques have greatly enhanced patient outcomes and quality of life, it is important to be aware of their drawbacks and possible adverse effects. To provide safe and effective healthcare interventions, a comprehensive and customized approach to therapy that takes into account each patient's particular needs is still essential.

CHAPTER FIVE

A HOLISTIC PERSPECTIVE ON HEALING

A holistic approach to healing recognizes the numerous connections between the physical, mental, and emotional elements of an individual's well-being and stresses the interconnectivity of these aspects. This viewpoint acknowledges that addressing a single issue in isolation could not result in full recovery. Rather, it promotes an all-encompassing and cohesive strategy that takes into account the individual as a whole.

THE VALUE OF A COMPREHENSIVE APPROACH

A holistic approach to healing is valuable because it takes into account the larger picture of a person's life. Through an analysis of an individual's emotional state, mental health, physical health, and even social circumstances, practitioners can gain a deeper understanding of the multifaceted nature of their illness.

This thorough knowledge makes it easier to create more individualized and efficient treatment programs that support general health and vitality rather than just symptom relief.

MIND-BODY LINK

A key idea in the holistic approach to healing is the mind-body link. It emphasizes how closely linked mental and physical health are, implying that one's condition has a direct impact on the other. For instance, bodily signs of stress could include headaches and tense muscles. On the other hand, persistent physical ailments can hurt mental health, resulting in psychological discomfort and worsening the general health issue. Identifying and treating this mind-body link is crucial to reaching the best possible health results.

Emotional health is critical to the holistic healing process when it comes to managing diseases like vulvodynia. Vulvodynia is a chronic pain condition that affects the vulvar area. Treating this issue involves a multifaceted strategy that takes into account the patient's mental well-being in addition to physical symptoms. Since pain perception and emotional health are intimately related, addressing the emotional components of vulvodynia can greatly reduce overall pain and enhance quality of life.

EMOTIONAL HEALTH IN THE MANAGEMENT OF VULVODYNIA

Recognizing and recognizing the potential emotional difficulties is a crucial part of managing emotional well-being in vulvodynia. Individuals who are in chronic pain frequently feel depressed, anxious, and frustrated. Incorporating techniques like mindfulness exercises, counseling, and support groups can provide you with important tools to deal with these emotional parts of life. Furthermore, establishing a therapeutic relationship between patients and healthcare professionals encourages an atmosphere in which emotional issues are freely shared and taken into account when developing a treatment plan.

A holistic approach to recovery highlights how intertwined mental, emotional, and physical healths are. This viewpoint emphasizes the value of treating emotional factors in disorders such as vulvodynia treatment and acknowledges the importance of the mind-body link. Adopting a holistic perspective on health enables professionals to provide more efficient and tailored care, encouraging not just the alleviation of symptoms but also general well-being for those in search of recovery and reconstruction.

CHAPTER SIX

ORGANIC SOLUTIONS

DIETARY MODIFICATIONS

The premise that our food intake has a significant impact on our general health is the foundation of the concept of dietary modifications as a natural cure. Maintaining a healthy, well-balanced diet is essential to assisting the body's inherent healing mechanisms. This entails arranging your meals to incorporate a range of fruits, vegetables, nutritious grains, and lean proteins. Stressing foods high in antioxidants, vitamins, and minerals can help to boost immunity and promote general health. To encourage the best possible digestion and nutritional absorption, dietary modifications may also entail modifying portion sizes and meal timings.

ANTI-INFLAMMATORY FOODS

Designed to address chronic inflammation, a prevalent cause of many health problems, anti-inflammatory foods are an important part of natural therapies. Nuts, seeds, olive oil, and fatty fish high in omega-3 fatty acids, including mackerel and salmon, are examples of these foods. Turmeric, berries, and leafy greens are also known to have anti-inflammatory qualities. The idea is to develop a diet that supports the body's healing process and lowers the risk of inflammatory-related illnesses by lowering inflammation.

FOODS TO AVOID

Natural cures include not only including healthy foods but also abstaining from specific toxins. Refined carbs, high sugar content, and highly processed foods can all exacerbate inflammation and have a detrimental effect on general health. People who are looking for natural solutions frequently avoid eating foods that include artificial additives and preservatives. Additionally, depending on personal sensitivity, some may decide to reduce or completely avoid common allergens like dairy or gluten.

HERBAL THERAPIES

Using plant-based solutions to treat a range of health issues is known as herbal therapy. For millennia, people from many cultures have used herbs for their possible medical benefits. This can involve adding herbs to tinctures, drinks, or supplements. Commonly utilized in herbal medicines are chamomile for relaxing, echinacea for immune support, and ginger for digestive problems. The goal of herbal therapy is frequently to enhance overall health by utilizing the therapeutic qualities of plants.

HERBS FOR PAIN RELIEF

Several herbs are well known for their inherent ability to reduce pain. For instance, turmeric includes curcumin, which is well-known for its anti-inflammatory and analgesic properties, while arnica has historically been applied topically to treat bruises and muscular aches. Herbs like aspirin and white willow bark both have salicin, which can be used as a pain reliever.

Including these herbs in one's routine—whether in the form of teas, salves, or supplements—can provide an alternative to traditional methods of managing pain.

LIFESTYLE CHANGES

Natural therapies may involve more extensive lifestyle changes than just nutritional adjustments. This may entail engaging in consistent physical activity to enhance general health and circulation. It is also stressed how important getting enough sleep is to the body's healing and restoration processes. It's usually advised to abstain from excessive alcohol and tobacco use because these substances might worsen inflammation and hurt health.

Stress management is important because stress is a constant in modern life and it can negatively impact one's physical and mental health. Natural stress-reduction solutions take a comprehensive approach, focusing on relaxation methods and lifestyle adjustments. Essential elements of stress management include eating a balanced diet, getting enough sleep, and exercising regularly. Furthermore, mindfulness activities like progressive muscular relaxation and deep breathing might help reduce stress. Herbal treatments, such as lavender aromatherapy or chamomile tea, are well-known for their relaxing effects and can be effective tools for naturally reducing stress.

EXERCISES FOR THE PELVIC FLOOR

Often referred to as Kegel exercises, these exercises are essential for maintaining pelvic health. By focusing on the muscles that support the pelvic organs, these exercises help prevent and treat conditions including pelvic organ prolapse and urine incontinence. Regular pelvic floor exercise improves bladder and bowel control by strengthening these muscles. These are great workouts for women to include in their routine, especially during pregnancy and after giving birth. Exercises for the pelvic floor not only treat particular health issues but also improve general core strength and stability.

ALTERNATIVE THERAPIES:

A wide variety of techniques that deviate from traditional medical methods fall under the umbrella of alternative therapies. Some find comfort in the holistic concepts of these therapies, while others regard them with mistrust. The goal of therapies like homeopathy, naturopathy, and herbal therapy is to assist the body's healing abilities. Identifying and treating underlying problems is generally given priority in alternative therapies as opposed to only treating symptoms. Those who are interested in these methods should investigate them under the supervision of licensed professionals, keeping in mind that individual differences can greatly affect how beneficial alternative therapies are.

ACUPUNCTURE

To promote energy flow, tiny needles are inserted into certain body sites during this age-old Chinese medical procedure. Acupuncture, which has its roots in the idea of balancing the body's essential energy, or qi, is used to treat a wide range of health issues. Acupuncture is praised for its ability to bring the body back into balance, and its benefits range from stress relief to managing chronic pain. Although the principles underlying acupuncture are still being better understood scientifically, many patients report beneficial results, highlighting acupuncture's importance as a supplementary therapy used in conjunction with traditional medical treatments.

YOGA AND MEDITATION

These age-old techniques, which have their roots in ancient traditions, are highly regarded for their ability to transform the body and mind. Yoga encourages flexibility, strength, and relaxation with its wide variety of physical postures (asanas) and breathing exercises (pranayama). Conversely, meditation promotes an elevated level of consciousness and attentiveness. When combined, these techniques promote a mind-body connection that benefits mental and physical health as well as stress reduction.

According to research, practicing yoga and meditation regularly can have a favorable effect on mental health by lowering anxiety, elevating mood, and building resilience overall. By incorporating these routines into daily life, one can foster long-term well-being and a sense of balance.

CHAPTER SEVEN

ESTABLISHING A NETWORK OF SUPPORT

THE VALUE OF ASSISTANCE

One of the most important components of resilience and personal well-being is creating a strong support network. It is impossible to overestimate the value of having a support network since it is essential for assisting people in overcoming hurdles, managing stress, and navigating life's problems. A network of people who offer emotional, practical, and occasionally financial help is referred to as a support system. This network could consist of coworkers, friends, mentors, relatives, and other people who provide a sense of understanding and connection.

GETTING ALONG WITH OTHERS

Humans need to connect fundamentally, and this connection is the foundation of a robust support network. Emotional health and a sense of belonging are enhanced by human relationships. People can share their ideas, emotions, and experiences through deep connections, which promotes empathy and understanding. These relationships reinforce the impression that one is not alone in enduring obstacles and serve as a buffer against the loneliness that frequently accompanies life's setbacks.

RESOURCES AND SUPPORT GROUPS

A comprehensive support system must include resources and support groups. Support groups provide a space for empathy and shared understanding by bringing people together who are going through comparable problems or experiences. Be it dealing with addiction, bereavement, health issues, or other life transitions, joining a support group offers a feeling of belonging and camaraderie. These organizations provide a forum for people to exchange ideas, coping mechanisms, and words of support.

Resources in a support system can also come in a variety of ways, from professional assistance to informational materials. With the right information, educational resources can provide people the power to better comprehend and navigate their surroundings. Professional assistance, like therapy or counseling, provides a controlled and private setting where people can examine their feelings, acquire understanding, and create coping skills.

It is very important to have a support system during uncertain or crises. It acts as a safety net, offering both practical and emotional support when needed most. A support system's capacity to work together can encourage people to overcome obstacles and develop resilience and adaptation.

The value of having a strong support network resides in its capacity to improve well-being, foster a feeling of community, and supply tools for resolving life's challenges. Developing a thorough and efficient support network is facilitated by establishing personal connections with people and actively utilizing resources and support groups.

CHAPTER EIGHT

FORMULATING A CUSTOMIZED STRATEGY

COLLABORATING WITH HEALTHCARE PROVIDERS

Developing a customized plan for one's health requires collaboration with healthcare providers. Collaboration in health management is encouraged when there is open and honest communication between healthcare providers and patients. It entails taking an active role in conversations on medical background, present symptoms, and lifestyle choices. Through this partnership, healthcare professionals can provide more individualized advice and support by gaining a thorough grasp of each patient's health situation.

A comprehensive evaluation conducted by medical specialists, nurses, and doctors starts the procedure. This evaluation takes into account the long-term objectives as well as the immediate concerns while evaluating the mental, emotional, and physical elements of health. It includes talking about current health issues, prescription drugs, dietary habits, allergies, and stress reduction techniques. This all-encompassing strategy guarantees that the customized plan takes into account each person's particular requirements and situation.

FORMULATING A COMPREHENSIVE THERAPY SCHEME

Creating a holistic treatment plan is essential to enhancing general well-being. Recognizing the interdependence of all facets of life, holistic health takes into account not just physical health but also mental, emotional, and social well-being.

A customized plan that takes a comprehensive approach could suggest adjustments to food, regular exercise, stress reduction methods, and mental health assistance. By combining these components, a comprehensive plan that takes into account the needs of the individual as a whole is ensured, encouraging long-lasting gains in health.

TRACKING DEVELOPMENT AND MODIFYING APPROACHES

Any customized plan's success depends on dynamic processes like tracking developments and making necessary strategy adjustments. Regular examinations and follow-ups with healthcare experts allow for the tracking of progress toward health goals. This continuing evaluation entails analyzing the effectiveness of adopted tactics, recognizing problems, and making appropriate improvements. Flexibility is key in adapting the plan to changing circumstances, ensuring that it remains relevant and effective over time. By regularly assessing and adjusting the plan, individuals can optimize their path to wellness and address any emerging health concerns.

Creating a personalized plan involves a collaborative effort with healthcare providers, acknowledging the importance of open communication and a comprehensive understanding of individual health. Developing a holistic treatment plan considers various aspects of well-being, promoting a balanced approach to health improvement. Monitoring progress and adjusting strategies are continuous processes that ensure the plan remains effective and adaptable to changing circumstances. Through these principles, individuals can embark on a journey toward optimal health and well-being.

ADVOCACY AND AWARENESS

Creating a personalized plan involves a thoughtful consideration of advocacy and awareness as integral components. Advocacy is the active promotion of a cause or principle, and incorporating it into a personal plan means identifying and championing issues that align with one's values. This can be achieved through various means, such as participating in community initiatives, joining advocacy groups, or leveraging social media platforms to raise awareness about specific issues. By integrating advocacy into a personal plan, individuals can contribute to positive change on a broader scale and foster a sense of purpose.

Awareness, on the other hand, entails a deep understanding of one's surroundings, personal strengths, and the socio-cultural context. Developing self-awareness is a crucial aspect of a personalized plan, as it enables individuals to make informed decisions aligned with their values and goals. Moreover, fostering awareness of broader societal issues is essential for cultivating empathy and a sense of responsibility toward collective well-being.

In the context of a personalized plan, advocacy and awareness work synergistically. For instance, an individual passionate about environmental issues may choose to advocate for sustainable practices in their community while raising awareness about the importance of conservation. This combination not only contributes to personal fulfillment but also creates a ripple effect, inspiring others to join the cause.

HOPE AND RESILIENCE

Hope and resilience are foundational elements in the construction of a personalized plan, serving as pillars that support individuals through challenges and uncertainties. Hope involves maintaining a positive outlook, setting optimistic goals, and believing in one's ability to overcome obstacles. Integrating hope into a personalized plan means cultivating a mindset that embraces possibilities and looks beyond setbacks. This can be achieved through practices such as setting realistic goals, visualizing success, and surrounding oneself with a supportive network.

Resilience, on the other hand, is the capacity to bounce back from adversity and adapt to change. In a personalized plan, resilience is cultivated by acknowledging that setbacks are a natural part of life and viewing them as opportunities for growth. Strategies for building resilience may include developing problem-solving skills, fostering social connections, and practicing self-care.

The symbiotic relationship between hope and resilience becomes evident in a personalized plan when faced with challenges. Individuals with a hopeful mindset are more likely to persevere, and their resilience allows them to navigate difficulties with a sense of purpose. This interplay enhances one's ability to learn from experiences, make necessary adjustments to the plan, and continue progressing toward personal goals.

Weaving advocacy and awareness into a personalized plan empowers individuals to contribute meaningfully to societal well-being, while the integration of hope and resilience provides the psychological fortitude needed to overcome challenges and pursue personal growth. Together, these concepts create a robust framework for individuals to lead purposeful and fulfilling lives.

www.ingramcontent.com/pod-product-compliance
Lightning Source LLC
Chambersburg PA
CBHW060848260726
48661CB00002B/671